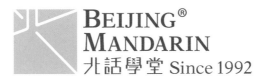

BEIJING® MANDARIN
北話學堂 Since 1992

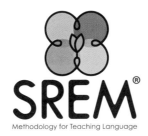

SREM®
Methodology for Teaching Language

Originated by BEIJING MANDARIN

**Laura WANG**
The Author

# MY FUN CHINESE
Preschool Textbook
READ & WRITE Series

## *I Can Read* (Textbook 3)

**Author**
Laura WANG
BEIJING MANDARIN

**Published by Beijing Mandarin (H.K.)**
11/F., Methodist House
36 Hennessy, Wanchai, Hong Kong
T (852) 2528 9319
E order@BeijingMandarin.com

**ISBN 978-988-12217-3-5**
© 2013 BEIJING MANDARIN
Hong Kong Library Publication Data

**Art Design**
LU Qun
**Illustration by**
WANG Chao, TAN Huabin
**Typeset by**
LU Qun, TAO Qingbin
**Cover Design**
LU Qun
**Design/Production**
Swank Cultural Innovation
Development Co., Ltd.

# 苗 乐 汉 语
学前课本　认写系列

## 我 会 认 ③

作　者　王丽琴
　　　　北话学堂

出　版　北话学堂 (H.K.)
　　　　香港湾仔轩尼诗道 36 号 1102 室

电　话　(852) 2528 9319
邮　箱　order@BeijingMandarin.com

国际书号　978–988–12217–3–5
© 2013 BEIJING MANDARIN
香港图书出版资料

美术设计　鲁　群
插　画　王　超　谭华斌
排　版　鲁　群　陶庆彬
封面设计　鲁　群
设计制作　尔雅文化创意发展有限公司

**MY FUN CHINESE - Preschool series**
Companion materials available

| | |
|---|---|
| *I Can Speak* | *Books 1-32* |
| *Oral Words 1-2-3* | *Daily Used Words* |
| *I Can Read* | *Books 1-6* |
| *I Can Write* | *Books 1-6* |
| *Characters 1-2-3* | *Basic Recognition* |

苗乐汉语 – 学前系列
配套书籍

| | |
|---|---|
| 我会说 | 1–32　册 |
| 基本语卡 | 日用高频词汇 |
| 我会认 | 1–6　册 |
| 我会写 | 1–6　册 |
| 基本字卡 | 笔画、偏旁、基本汉字 |

# I Can Read Chinese Radicals

*wǒ    huì    rèn*

# 我 会 认

**3**

## 41 Basic Chinese Radicals & Basic Characters

## 41基本偏旁和独体字

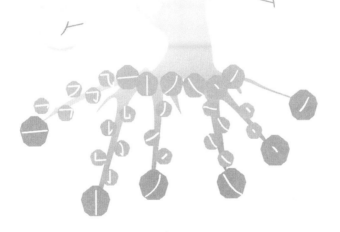

Student's Name

学 生 姓 名 _____

# Contents
## 目 录

# 41 Basic Radicals & Basic Characters
## 个基本偏旁和独体字

1. The 6 Basic Strokes and their Transformed Strokes make up Radicals and Basic Characters.

2. Radicals and Basic Characters make up all Chinese Characters.

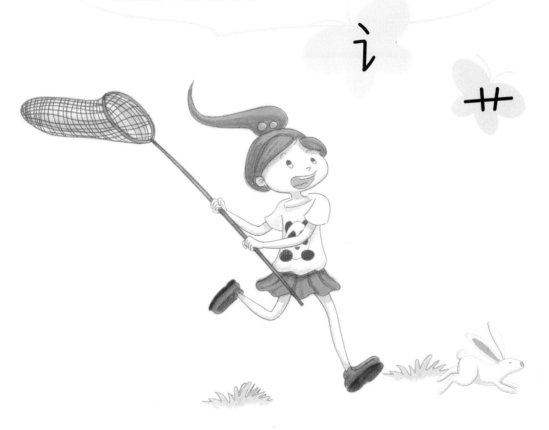

**1. 6 Basic Strokes and their Transformed Strokes**

| 6 Basic Strokes | Transformed Strokes | | | | |
|---|---|---|---|---|---|
| ① 一 héng Horizontal | ¬ | ﬁ | ㄱ | ㄱ | ㄟ |
| ② 丨 shù Vertical | ↓ | ↓ | ) | ㄴ | ㄴ |
| ③ 丿 piě Left-falling | ノ | ノ | ) | | |
| ④ ㇏ nà Right-falling | ＼ | ＼ | ㇄ | ～ | |
| ⑤ 丶 diǎn Dot | 丶 | ＼ | | | |
| ⑥ ㇀ tí Rising | | | | | |

2

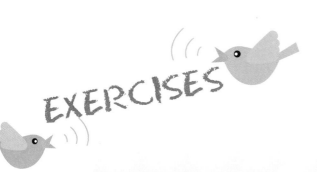

# EXERCISES

Can you read aloud the 6 Basic Strokes?

Can you trace all Strokes with your finger?

Can you memorize all Strokes by heart well?

## 2. 6 Basic Strokes and their Transformed Strokes make up Radicals and Basic Characters

*Should remember:* **1**

Radicals have their meanings, but they cannot be read out and cannot be used alone.

For example:

Basic Characters have their meanings. And they can be read out, can be used alone and can be used as radicals in other characters. **2**

丿

ice

For example:

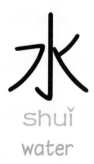

shuǐ
water

### 3. Radicals and Basic Characters make up all Chinese Characters

*Should remember:*

Basically, all Chinese Characters are made by Radicals and Basic Characters.

For example:

冫
ice

水
shuǐ
water

冰
bīng
ice

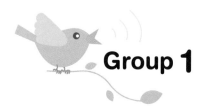

# Group 1

**Basic Radical**

1

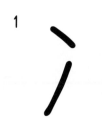

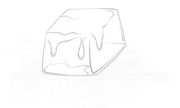

**Basic Radical**

2

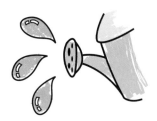

**Basic Radical**

3

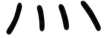

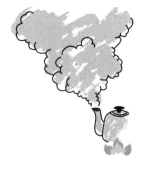

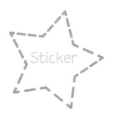

**Basic Radical**

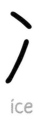

ice

**Basic Character**

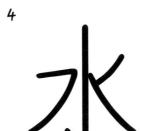

**Basic Radical**

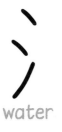

water

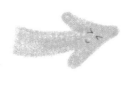

shuǐ

water

**Basic Radical**

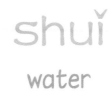

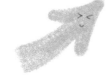

heat

## Exercises
## 练习

● **Find out Radical from the character group, then copy it in the box and write down its meaning**
找出每组汉字的偏旁，然后把它和它的意思写在方格里

冰　冷
凉　次

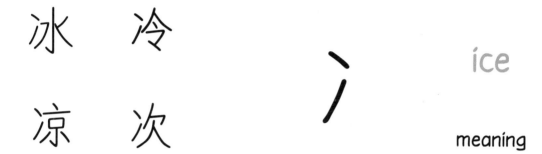

*ice*

meaning

没　汁
洗　游

meaning

8

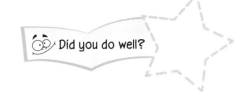

点 黑

热 然

meaning

**Find out Basic Character "水", then copy it in the box and write down its meaning**

找出"水"字，然后把它和它的意思写在方格里

我要喝水。

meaning

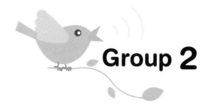

# Group 2

Basic Radical

5

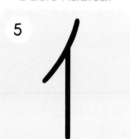

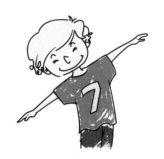

Basic Radical

6

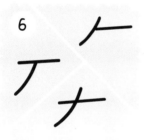

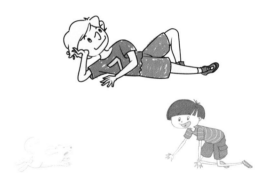

Basic Radical

7

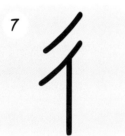

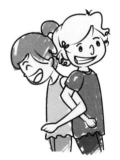

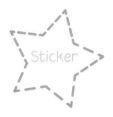

*Basic Radical*

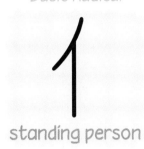

standing person

*Basic Radical*

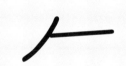

sleeping person

*Basic Radical*

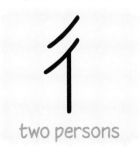

two persons

**Basic Character**

8

人

rén

person

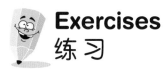

## Exercises
练习

● **Find out Radical from the character group, then copy it in the box and write down its meaning**
找出每组汉字的偏旁，然后把它和它的意思写在方格里

你 他 们 什 伯

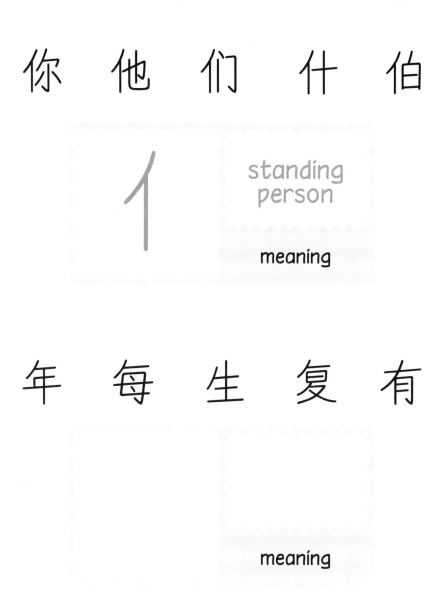

亻

standing person

meaning

年 每 生 复 有

meaning

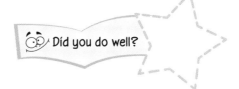

很　得　行　往

meaning

● **Find out Basic Character "人", then copy it in the box and write down its meaning**
找出"人"字，然后把它和它的意思写在方格里

一人有一口。

meaning

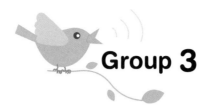

# Group **3**

Basic Radical

9

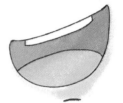

Basic Radical

10

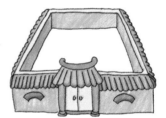

Basic Radical

11

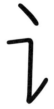

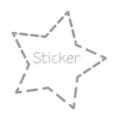

*Basic Radical*

mouth

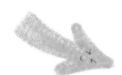

*Basic Radical*

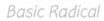

big place

*Basic Radical*

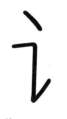

talk, speak

**Basic Character**

12

kǒu

mouth

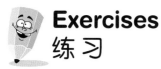 **Exercises**
练习

● **Find out Radical from the character group, then copy it in the box and write down its meaning**
找出每组汉字的偏旁，然后把它和它的意思写在方格里

问　　吃　　喝　　唱

mouth

meaning

回　　国　　元　　囚

meaning

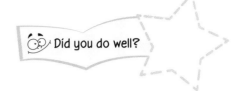

说　请　让　认

meaning

● **Find out Basic Character "口", then copy it in the box and write down its meaning**
找出"口"字，然后把它和它的意思写在方格里

一　人　有　一　口。

meaning

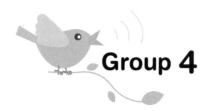

# Group 4

*Basic Radical*

13

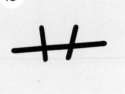

*Basic Radical*

14

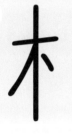

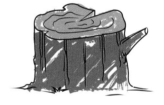

*Basic Radical*

15

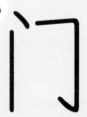

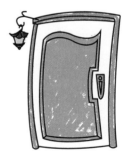

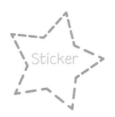

**Character**

**Basic Radical**

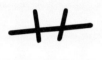

grass

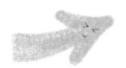

草

cǎo
grass

**Basic Radical**

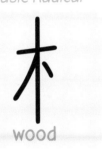

wood

**Basic Character**

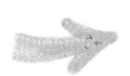

16

木

mù
wood

**Basic Radical**

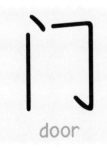

door

**Basic Character**

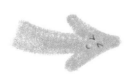

17

门

mén
door

19

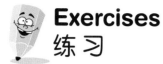
**Exercises**
练习

● **Find out Radical from the character group, then copy it in the box and write down its meaning**
找出每组汉字的偏旁，然后把它和它的意思写在方格里

草　花

节　开

艹

grass

meaning

木　椅

床　树

meaning

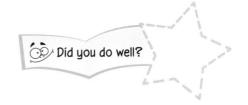
Did you do well?

门　闷

阔　闲

meaning

● **Find out Character "草", then copy it in the box and write down its meaning**
找出"草"字, 然后把它和它的意思写在方格里

小羊吃草。

meaning

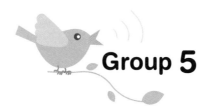

# Group 5

Basic Radical

18

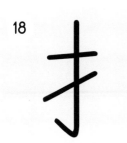

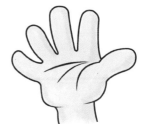

Basic Radical

19

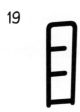

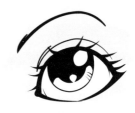

Basic Radical

20

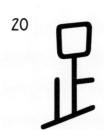

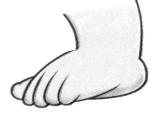

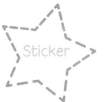

Sticker

**Basic Character**

21

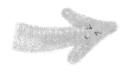

手

shǒu
hand

*Basic Radical*

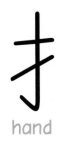

hand

*Basic Radical*

eye

**Basic Character**

22

目

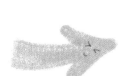

mù
eye

*Basic Radical*

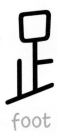

foot

**Basic Character**

23

足

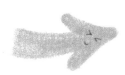

zú
foot

**Exercises**
练习

● **Find out Radical from the character group, then copy it in the box and write down its meaning**
找出每组汉字的偏旁，然后把它和它的意思写在方格里

打　找

拍　把

扌

hand

meaning

目　眼

晴　看

meaning

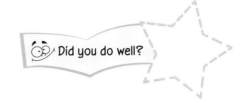

跳　跑

路　足

meaning

● **Find out Basic Character "手", then copy it in the box and write down its meaning**
找出"手"字，然后把它和它的意思写在方格里

左手和右手。

meaning

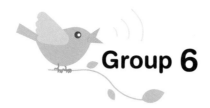

# Group 6

*Basic Radical*

24

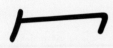

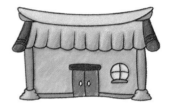

*Basic Radical*

25

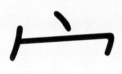

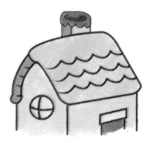

*Basic Radical*

26

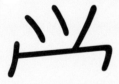

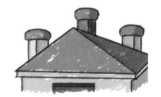

Sticker

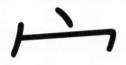    roof

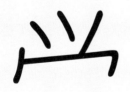    roof with
a chimney

roof with
three chimneys

## Exercises
练习

● **Find out Radical from the character group, then copy it in the box and write down its meaning**
找出每组汉字的偏旁，然后把它和它的意思写在方格里

欠　次

欢　歌

⌐　roof

meaning

字　家

完　安

meaning

28

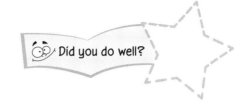
学　觉

meaning

**Find out Basic Character "家", then copy it in the box and write down its meaning**
找出"家"字，然后把它和它的意思写在方格里

我有一个家。

meaning

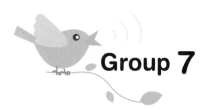

# Group 7

*Basic Radical*

27

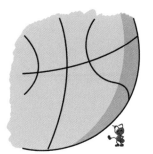

*Basic Radical*

28

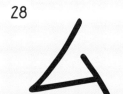

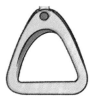

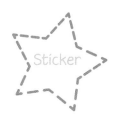

*Basic Radical*

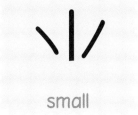

small

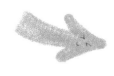

**Basic Character**

29

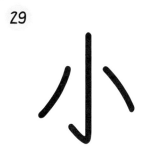

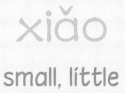

xiǎo

small, little

*Basic Radical*

triangle

## Exercises
练习

● **Find out Radical from the character group, then copy it in the box and write down its meaning**
找出每组汉字的偏旁，然后把它和它的意思写在方格里

小　少

尖　当

small

meaning

么　去

台　能

meaning

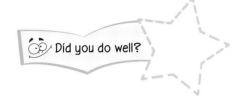

● **Find out Basic Character "小", then copy it in the box and write down its meaning**
找出"小"字，然后把它和它的意思写在方格里

# 我有小牛。

meaning

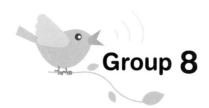

# Group 8

*Basic Radical*

30

力

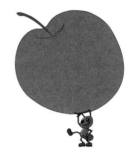

*Basic Radical*

31

女

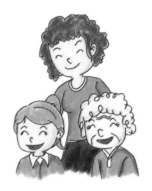

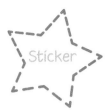

**Basic Character**

32

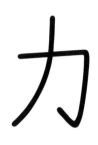

*Basic Radical*

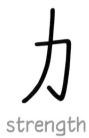 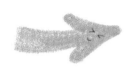

strength

lì
strength

**Basic Character**

33

*Basic Radical*

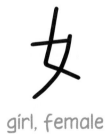 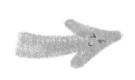 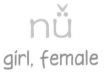

girl, female

nǚ
girl, female

## Exercises
练习

● **Find out Radical from the character group, then copy it in the box and write down its meaning**
找出每组汉字的偏旁，然后把它和它的意思写在方格里

男　力

功　加

| 力 | strength |
|---|---|
| | meaning |

妈　她

姐　妹

| | |
|---|---|
| | meaning |

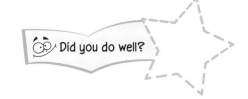

● **Find out Basic Character "力", then copy it in the box and write down its meaning**
找出"力"字, 然后把它和它的意思写在方格里

小牛有力。

meaning

● **Find out Basic Character "女", then copy it in the box and write down its meaning**
找出"女"字, 然后把它和它的意思写在方格里

一男一女。

meaning

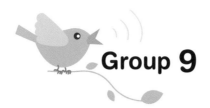

# Group 9

Basic Radical

34

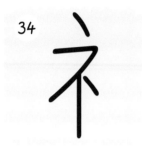

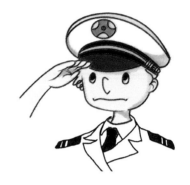

Basic Radical

35

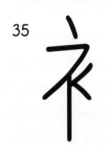

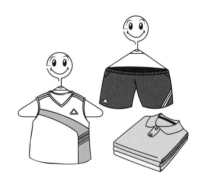

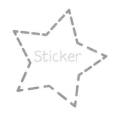

*Basic Radical*

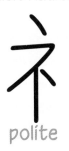

polite

*Basic Radical*

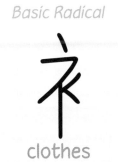

clothes

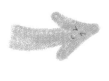

### Basic Character

36

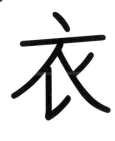

yī
clothes

**Exercises**
练习

● **Find out Radical from the character group, then copy it in the box and write down its meaning**
找出每组汉字的偏旁，然后把它和它的意思写在方格里

祝　礼

福　神

礻 polite

meaning

被　裙

裤　袜

meaning

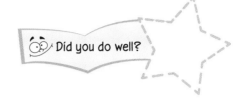

**Find out Basic Character "礼", then copy it in the box and write down its meaning**
找出"礼"字，然后把它和它的意思写在方格里

人人有礼。

meaning

**Find out Basic Character "衣", then copy it in the box and write down its meaning**
找出"衣"字，然后把它和它的意思写在方格里

有衣有食。

meaning

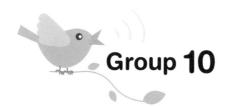

# Group **10**

*Basic Radical*

37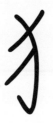

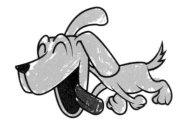

*Basic Radical*

38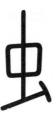

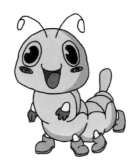

*Basic Radical*

39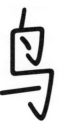

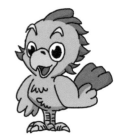

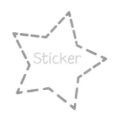

*Basic Radical*

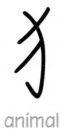

animal

**Basic Character**

40

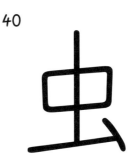

chóng
caterpillar
worm

*Basic Radical*

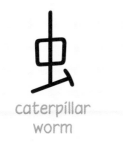

caterpillar
worm

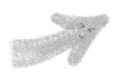

**Basic Character**

41

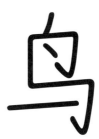

*Basic Radical*

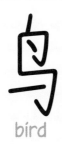

bird

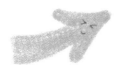

niǎo
bird

**Exercises**
练习

● **Find out Radical from the character group, then copy it in the box and write down its meaning**
找出每组汉字的偏旁，然后把它和它的意思写在方格里

虫　虽

虾　蛇

虫　worm

meaning

狗　猫

狮　猴

meaning

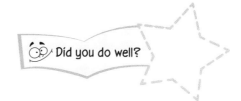

鸟　鸡

鸭　鹅

meaning

**Find out Basic Character "鸟", then copy it in the box and write down its meaning**
找 出 "鸟" 字, 然 后 把 它 和 它 的 意 思 写 在 方 格 里

鸟 在 天 上 飞。

meaning

# Conclusion
# 总 结

● **Read aloud and remember the following**
读一读，记一记

 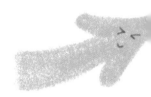

Radicals have their meanings, but they cannot be read out and cannot be used alone.

 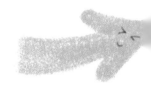

Basic Characters have their meanings. And they can be read out, can be used alone and can be used as Radicals in other characters.

 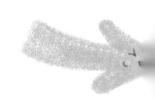

Radicals and the Basic Characters are often puzzled into Chinese Characters to indicate the meanings of the Characters.

 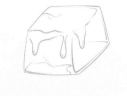

ice

Radical

shuǐ

water

 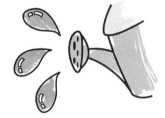

Basic Character

bīng

ice

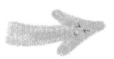 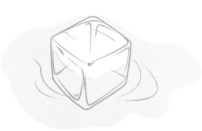

Character

Did you do well?

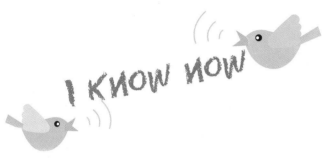

1. Basically, all Chinese Characters are made by Radicals and Basic Characters.

2. Radicals and Basic Characters are made by the 6 Basic Strokes and their Transformed Strokes.

# 2 Revision
## 复习

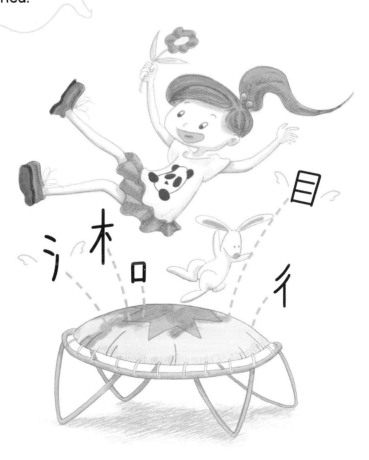

I like to review what
I have learned.

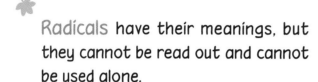Radicals have their meanings, but they cannot be read out and cannot be used alone.

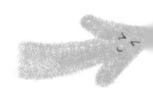

Basic Characters have their meanings. And they can be read out, can be used alone and can be used as Radicals in other characters.

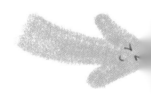

Radicals and the Basic Characters are often puzzled into Chinese Characters to indicate the meanings of the Characters.

ice

Radical

 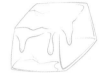

水

shuǐ
water

Basic Character

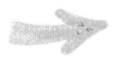 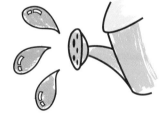

冰

bīng
ice

Character

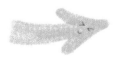 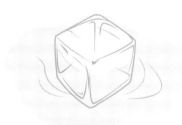

**Connect the Radical and the Basic Character to its picture**
把偏旁或汉字和对应的图片连起来

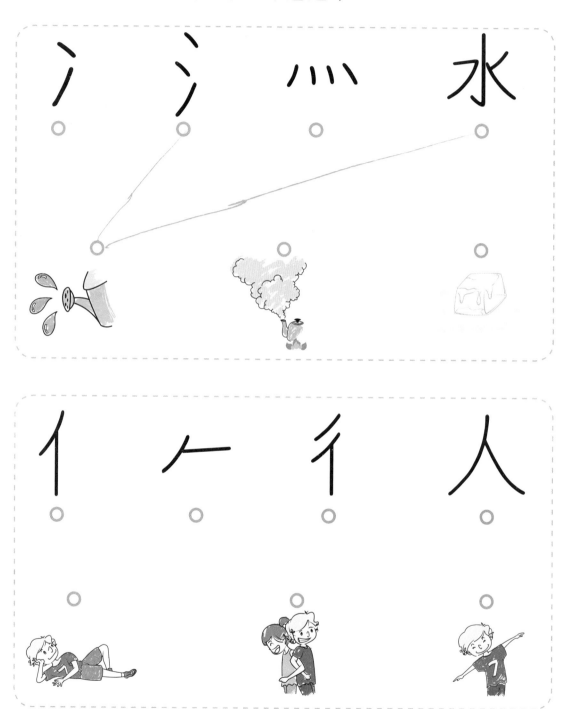

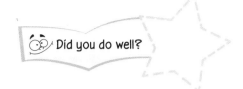
Did you do well?

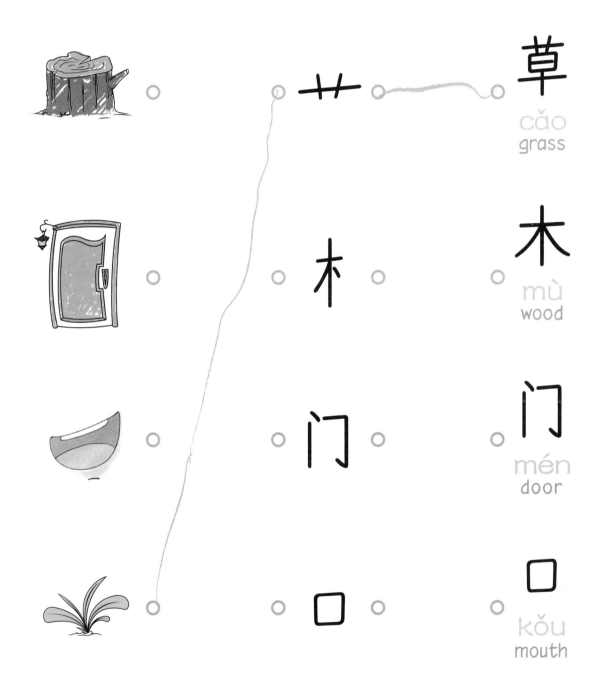

草
cǎo
grass

木
mù
wood

门
mén
door

口
kǒu
mouth

**Look at the Basic Characters and the Radicals, draw a picture for them**
看看偏旁和独体字，然后为它们画图

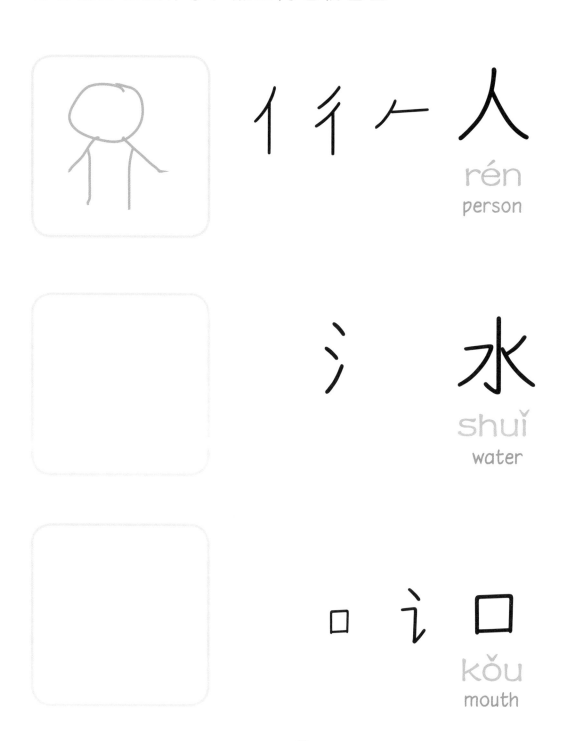

亻 彳 亻 人
rén
person

氵 水
shuǐ
water

口 讠 口
kǒu
mouth

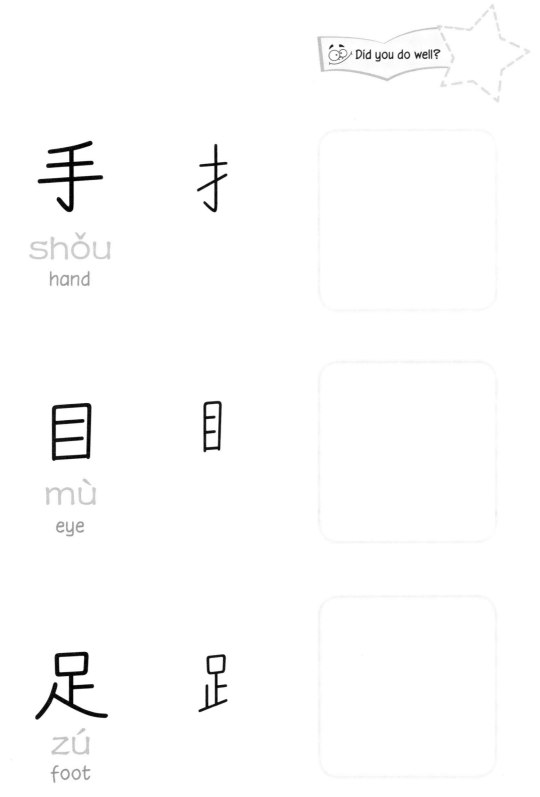

手　扌

shǒu
hand

目　目

mù
eye

足　𧾷

zú
foot

## Connect the Radical or the Basic Character to its picture
把偏旁或汉字和对应的图片连起来

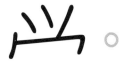  ○    ○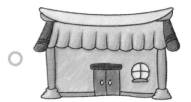

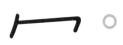  ○    ○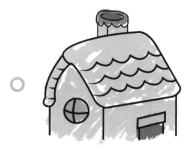

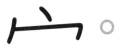  ○    ○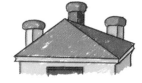

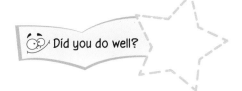
Did you do well?

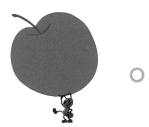

力

○　○

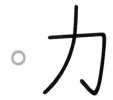

小

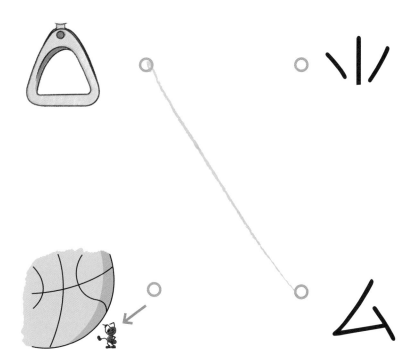

ム

**Draw a picture for the Radical and write down its meaning**
画 出 偏 旁 或 独 体 字 , 然 后 写 出 英 文 意 思

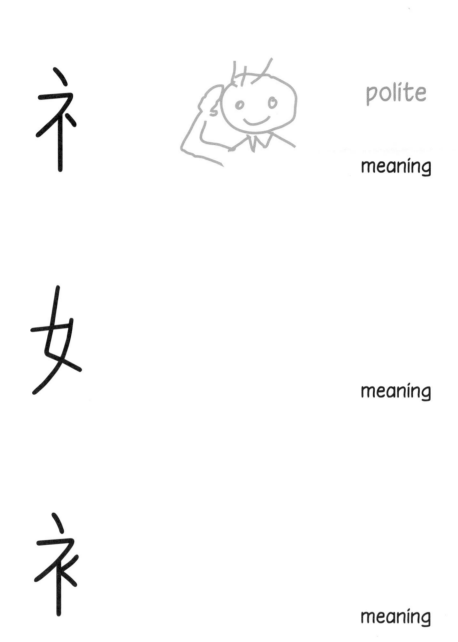

礻                    polite

                    meaning

女

                    meaning

衤

                    meaning

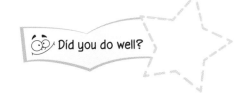
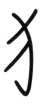

meaning

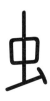

meaning

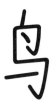

meaning

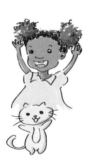

## *Grateful Acknowledgement*
## *is awarded to*

**Professor Liu Xun**
北京语言大学
Beijing Language and Culture University

**Chief Editor Ms. Hou Ming**
三联（香港）出版社
Joint Publishing (H.K.) Co., Ltd.

**Director Mr. Duke**
尔雅文化创意发展有限公司
Swank Cultural Innovation Development Co., Ltd.

Their constructive criticism, thoughtful suggestion and continual support are invaluable for the success of writing and publishing these books.

## *Grateful Recognition*
## *is given to*

**Mr. Richard C. K. Wong**
Honorary Chancellor

**Mr. Nadjib Hermanto**
Independent Management Consultant

for their long time friendship, encouragement, invaluable advice and guidance.

**Laura WANG**
The Author